Herbal Remedies & Solutions: An Introduction to the Benefits of Herbal Remedies

Simple Herbal Solutions for Common Ailments

By: Melanie Watlings

9781630225827

I0423648

TABLE OF CONTENTS

Melanie Watlings

Publishers Notes

Speedy Publishing LLC

40 E. Main St., #1156

Newark, DE 19711

www.speedypublishing.co

Cover Artwork: 24 Hr. Designs Ltd.

Editing: Speedy Publishing LLC

Book design: Speedy Publishing LLC

ISBN: 9781630225827

This is a reprint book.

DISCLAIMER

This publication is intended to provide helpful and informative material. It is not intended to diagnose, treat, cure, or prevent any health problem or condition, nor is intended to replace the advice of a physician. No action should be taken solely on the contents of this book. Always consult your physician or qualified health-care professional on any matters regarding your health and before adopting any suggestions in this book or drawing inferences from it.

The author and publisher specifically disclaim all responsibility for any liability, loss or risk, personal or otherwise, which is incurred as a consequence, directly or indirectly, from the use or application of any contents of this book.

Any and all product names referenced within this book are the trademarks of their respective owners. None of these owners have sponsored, authorized, endorsed, or approved this book.

Always read all information provided by the manufacturers' product labels before using their products. The author and publisher are not responsible for claims made by manufacturers.

DEDICATION

This book is dedicated to Jackie for turning me on to taking better care of my body without the use of chemical drugs. Thank you so much!

INTRODUCTION

Herbal remedies are milder than traditional medicines and have fewer side effects, and most are very safe if used as directd.

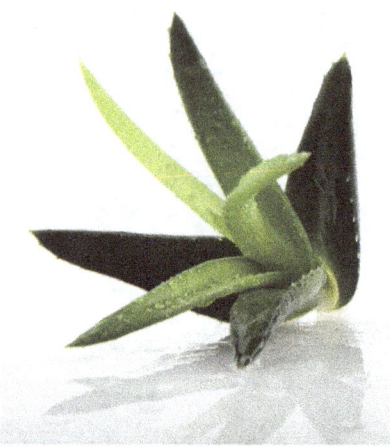

Herbs are plants used in medicine. Natural healing has come to denote any type of natural means used to aid in healing. Although most herbal remedies are from plants, there are some that are mineral or animal products as well. Herbal medicine is also called phytotherapy, the science of using herbal remedies to treat illnesses.

People have been using herbs for hundreds of years to treat all types of illnesses and symptoms. Throughout history we can find examples from many cultures of their use of herbal remedies. The ancient Egyptians used herbs in healing and in ceremonies as well. There are hieroglyphics that depict the use of herbs on some ancient walls. In ancient China, herbs were an important part of healing and still are used in traditional Chinese medicine.

Today, more and more people are turning to herbal remedies to cure anything from headaches to skin conditions to colds. You can find an herbal cure for just about anything that ails you. There are also herbal remedies that are used as preventions for many types of illnesses as well.

Medical doctors are also getting involved in more natural cures. There are specific additional medical courses available that instruct on herbal cures and their uses. A holistic M.D. is a licensed physician who has completed not only the traditional medical studies, but has additional education in the philosophy and methods of natural healing. A N.D is a doctor of naturopathic medicine, and they are recognized and licensed in a number of states.

Herbalists understand how herbs act to treat certain ailments in the body. The body is like a small ecosystem unto itself, and everything is balanced just right. When some part of the body becomes unbalanced, herbs can be used to help restore balance again.

Usually, herbal remedies are milder than traditional medicines and have fewer side effects, and most are very safe if used as directed. The body can build up a resistance to some medications, such as antibiotics, when they are used too much. Herbal cures are helpful when treating illnesses that are not too serious. There are many ways to use herbs as effective treatments.

CHAPTER 1- CHOOSING HERBAL PRODUCTS

Herbal products should be selected based on the problem that is being experienced.

There are many herbal products and cures available. With the advent of more and more natural food stores, more herbal goods are commonly accessible. Herbs are used in many types of products, and they can be taken orally or used topically. Specific herbs have specific uses or cures associated with them. These are uses that have come to be known over years of use and handed down from generation to generation.

In recent times, scientific studies have been done which prove that certain herbal cures work for specific illnesses.

Topical herbal remedies are available in several forms. These are forms used for external use.

Salve - Salves are healing preparations that are applied to the skin. They are generally thick creams that last a long time on the skin, helping to keep moisture in. Salves have protective qualities that shield the skin from harsh effects of sun and wind. Popular salves are those made with calendula, St. John's wort and comfrey.

Poultice - A poultice is a traditional preparation of fresh or dried whole herbs. The herbs are mashed into a pasty consistency and applied topically to the affected area. Herbs can be moistened and heated and then applied to the skin. Poultices are the way your great-grandmother would have applied herbs and it's still a useful method today. A crude method, poultices are great for instant use and can use parts of the plant that aren't normally used, such as the root and stems.

Compress - A compress is similar to a poultice. Fresh or dried herbs are mashed and combined with water to make a paste. The paste is then applied to the skin or put into a small bundle, often in fabric, to be held against the skin.

Oils - Infused oils are made by combining herbs with oil, usually extra-virgin olive oil, and heated on a slow heat. The mixture is then steeped for at least two weeks, then strained and put into jars. Oils can be used for skin irritations and is commonly used as massage oil.

Ointment - Similar to salves, ointments are thicker in consistency. They are used topically on the skin and are particularly good for minor skin irritations and burns.

Ingestible herbal remedies are taken orally. These include various forms.

Infusions - Infusions are the most common way that people take herbal remedies. An infusion is a preparation that uses water as a solvent to mix with crude botanicals. The mixture may start out hot or can be a cold mixture. Usually, hot water mixtures infuse the herbs more readily and are therefore made hot and then cooled down for use. The mixture is steeped, rather than boiled. That is, it is let to set in the hot water for a period of time, depending on the type of herbs that are used. Infusions are generally the weakest of the herbal preparations.

Decoction - A decoction is similar to an infusion because water is used. However, a decoction uses water to boil the herbs and then squeezes them into a container. That "juice" is more concentrated than an infusion and is twice as potent. In prepared decoctions, alcohol is used as a preservative. Otherwise, the decoction would spoil rapidly. Decoctions are often used as additives in prepared foods or drinks.

Tincture - Similar to decoctions, tinctures are prepared by allowing herbs to sit in liquids for long periods of time to solubilize them. Herbs are stored for weeks to months in dark glass containers containing an ingredient that will make them soluble. That may be water, vinegar, alcohol or glycerine. The herbs break down in the liquid and dissolve. The remaining mixture is strained or pressed. Tinctures are often used added to foods or drinks.

Syrup - Similar to tinctures, syrups are a thicker liquid. These are most often taken alone as a remedy. Syrups generally have higher concentrations of herbs and care should be taken to follow the directions properly.

Tea - There are a number of pre-made herbal teas on the market these days. There are also tea bags that come in a variety of herbal mixtures. These are so common that they are available at any regular supermarket. Tea is actually a form of infusion.

Capsules or Tablets - Next to infusions, capsules are the next most common way to take herbs. Supplements are available in tablet form for almost any herb known. These are ingested in the same way you take aspirin. They dissolve in the stomach and get into your body.

When you are choosing herbal products there are some things to keep in mind. First, make sure you understand what you want the product to do. Read the label. Sometimes there are additional ingredients that may be unnecessary for your ailment. Always choose a product that most closely identifies with your disorder.

Smell the product. That will tell you how much of the herb is actually in the product. This is especially true with creams and salves. If you can't smell the herb chances are there is not enough of it in the product to help you. Because herbal products are not governed the same way as food products, the user must take more caution in purchasing and using these items. Check for an expiration date on the item.

To keep herbal products good always store them in a cool, dry area. Also, try to store them in a dark area. Light often will break down the mixture and will change the strength. Many products come in dark containers to help keep light from affecting the products.

If you have herbal products that you haven't used in a while, always smell them before using them. If they smell rancid, they have probably gone bad. Although this won't affect the topical cures, you certainly don't want to ingest herbal mixtures of questionable freshness. Most products manufactured by large companies have a long shelf life. However, homemade products may last only weeks to several months. Keep homemade products in the refrigerator to make them keep longer.

Know what you're taking and why. Even though the products are herbal and natural does not mean that they are all safe. Interactions can occur and you should be aware of these possible interactions before taking any herbal remedy.

Purchase your herbal products from a reputable source. Health food stores and many drug stores carry herbal products. Your local health food store will be able to answer many of your questions as they are trained in this area. If you buy herbal products over the Internet, be sure that the company is reputable. The FDA or any other agency does not control herbal products, so the quality can vary greatly between brands.

CHAPTER 2- HOW TO USE AROMATHERAPY

Although aromatherapy does not claim to cure any diseases, it helps to soothe the body and mind in many ways.

Aromatherapy uses herbal oils to treat the mental, emotional and physical properties of an illness through the sense of smell. Herbs are fragrant and give off particular scents that each have properties thought to help heal certain illnesses. Aromatherapy is thought to be especially helpful to calm nerves and soothe anxiety.

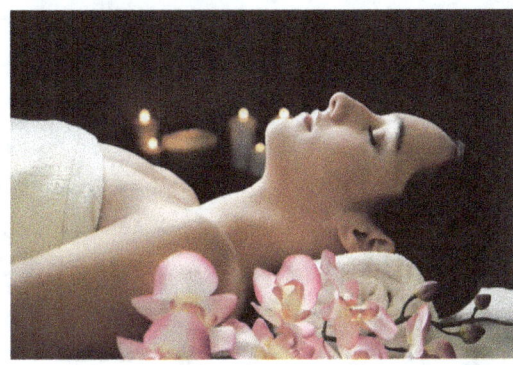

Aromatherapy was used in prehistoric times, and has been used throughout history ever since. Incense is a form of aromatherapy that has been popular for centuries in many cultures. Today, the use of aromatherapy is popular to help promote health and well being and to reduce the effects of stress.

Aromatherapy works by releasing herb infused oils or liquids into the air. Essential oils may be placed onto a small cloth and then placed where the aroma can disperse throughout the area. Aromatherapy has become a popular and accepted method in the last several decades, and products are now widely available at local stores and supermarkets. Aromatherapy is used in many bath products and lotions. Examples of aromatherapy products include air fresheners or diffusers, as well as electric and battery powered products that spread the scent through the use of small fans.

Aromatherapy is a holistic approach to healing, taking into consideration the needs of the whole person. This takes into consideration your physical, mental and emotional states to help determine which essential oils are best suited for your particular situation. Aromatherapists mix essential oils together to create blends that are specific to your needs.

Your sense of smell is the only sense that actually has nerve receptors exposed outside the body. When a scent is detected special messages are transported to the limbic system inside the brain to be processed. The scent is identified there. This part of the brain also stores memories, which is why certain smells are often strongly associated with certain memories in your life. Blending essential oils together can form scents that are pleasant and relaxing, thus helping to reduce and eliminate stress and tension.

Essential oils are usually dissolved in either a water or oil base to blend together. The amounts used are small and do not cause any potential danger in these extremely low doses. These blends are often available as pre-made mixtures and are also able to be custom blended by an aromatherapist or by you at home.

Massage therapy uses aromatherapy to help in relaxation. Essential oils are used to massage the body. Besides the scent of the massage oil, small amounts of essential oils can also enter the body through the skin into the bloodstream. Again, these small doses are not considered harmful.

Although aromatherapy does not claim to cure any diseases, it is, nonetheless, responsible for helping soothe the body and mind in many ways. It can help improve your mood and general feelings of well-being. Specific combinations of essential oils can help create euphoric sensations in the brain. Aromatherapy can improve blood circulation and also improve lymphatic function when combined with massage therapy. Some soothing herbs are now used in common baby products to calm and help lessen the effects of colic and to help promote better sleep.

Many herbs are used, and here are some of the most common herbs that are used in essential oils for aromatherapy.

Lavender - Lavender helps relieve tired muscles and can actually reduce muscle spasms. It is a very safe herb and is often used in many items, especially in baby products because of its gentle nature. There are relatively no side effects from using lavender. It is often used to calm anxiety and helps in eliminating insomnia. A diluted version is often used in a spray that can be used on beds and pillows to promote sleep. It is often used in small pillows that can be heated in the microwave and then applied onto the neck and back muscles to help relax them. Lavender blends well with most other herbs, making it a perfect choice for many herbal mixtures.

Bergamot - Bergamot is very uplifting. It is often used to help depression or mood swings. It is also helpful in eliminating insomnia and is said to help stop nightmares from occurring. It is a mild herb and is unlikely to cause any ill effects. It mixes well with most other herbs, including lavender, cedarwood, rosemary, geranium and lemongrass.

Tea Tree - Tea tree oil is an herb that is often used in topical mixtures to help fight bacterial infections. Used in aromatherapy, tea tree is said to help promote energy and helps relieve anxiety. It is also used to help aid in poor concentration. Another mild herb, tea tree is not associated with any known side effects and is safe to use. It mixes well with eucalyptus, bergamot, lavender and peppermint.

Neroli - Neroli is often used to help control the signs of stress and anxiety. Long used as a remedy, neroli is known to help those with exhaustion feel better and more relaxed. It helps with panic disorders and is said to calm fears, insomnia, and moodiness. It was used for many years as a treatment for grieving widows as it helps calm and soothe the mind. Neroli is a mild and safe treatment, and it blends well with most other herbs, including ylang-ylang, jasmine, melissa and peppermint.

Melissa - Melissa is known for its antiseptic properties when used on the skin. In aromatherapy, melissa is known to ease panic attacks. It is also used to help those who are overcoming addictions with alcohol or tobacco, as it helps alleviate those cravings. Melissa helps encourage calmness and brings serenity to you, and helps stop fear and depression. It mixes well with most other herbs, especially jasmine, neroli, geranium, and chamomile. Melissa in aromatherapy is mild, but when used on the skin it can cause irritation for those with sensitive skin. Test a small spot on the skin prior to use.

Frankincense - Frankincense has been used for thousands of years and has strong religious associations to the Bible. It is a popular herb used to help restore confidence and calm. It helps calm fears and paranoia, as well as nightmares. It helps restore balance to those who have signs of emotional exhaustion. It is mild and is unlikely to cause any adverse reactions, and mixes well with most other herbs, including ylang-ylang, myrrh, neroli, melissa, cedarwood, rosemary and lavender.

Juniper - Juniper is commonly grown in the United States as well as Europe. The berries are very pungent and are used in the making of gin. Juniper is used to clear and stimulate the mind, and is said to prevent worry and unpleasant memories. It can renew enthusiasm and give you a new zest for life. It is safe as an aromatic; however, you should use caution when ingesting it if you have any kidney disease. Juniper blends well with most other herbs such as lavender, frankincense, tea tree and jasmine.

Herbs can be used in aromatherapy treatments in several ways. Essential oils are the easiest to use. These are made by distilling the plant material and mixing with a small amount of liquid or oil. Essential oils are concentrated and need to be diluted when used, and a few drops are all that is necessary when mixing with other oils. Essential oils can be used in baths, in lotions and perfumes and as inhalations. They are readily available at most health food or natural stores, as well as online. Do not put essential oils directly on the skin without first diluting them. These concentrations are strong and even safe herbs can cause irritations if not diluted. Be sure to dilute even more when using with young children.

Chapter 3- Symptoms Guide

Specific herbs can be combined to treat certain ailments from the common cold to arthritis. It is important to have the remedies prepared by a licensed herbologist.

Herbal Remedies A-F

Here is a list of common ailments, and the herbal remedies that are often used to combat them. If you have been diagnosed with a certain disease or disorder, you may be able to try an herbal remedy.

Make sure you check with a doctor or herbalist if you are already taking a prescription drug, because certain prescription drugs can have interactions with herbal remedies. Also, do not substitute herbal cures for prescription medications unless your doctor has cleared you to do so.

Certain ailments, such as heart problems, require specific continued doses of prescription medication. If you are currently being treated by a physician for a medical problem and you would like to try an herbal remedy, consult your doctor. Explain your desire to try to treat your condition with herbal remedies and ask for his help in figuring out how best to go about it.

That being said, many herbal cures are available for common ailments, especially those you don't normally see a doctor for, such as sunburn and upset stomach. Many herbal remedies are safe to use if you are not already on a prescription drug.

Acne

Some acne usually occurs in teenagers, although many adults have occasional bouts of acne as well. There are many factors that contribute to acne. Keratin is a protein that is produced by the skin cells, and too much of it can form clumps that block oil ducts. When this happens, bacteria can form, causing a pimple. Another possible cause of acne in teen girls is hormonal changes. Other theories about acne have little foundation to back them up. For example, certain foods have been said to cause acne, such as chocolate or French fries. These claims are unfounded. There is no evidence that foods cause acne. There are drug treatments available for the treatment of acne. The most common are topical treatments, which often contain antibiotics.

Herbal Remedies For Acne Include:

Tea Tree Oil - Tea tree oil comes from this Australian tree. Used as a topical treatment, in studies it was found to be as effective as benzoil peroxide but with fewer side effects. To use, first gently cleanse the skin and pat dry. Apply diluted tea tree oil to the problem areas and let dry. You can purchase tea tree oil already diluted or you can dilute yourself using jojoba oil with 5 to 15% tea tree oil. Use the mixture twice a day. Test a small spot first to ensure that you do not get a rash. Some people with sensitive skin can have a small reaction to tea tree oil. Do not take internally.

Lavender - Lavender essential oil is often used as an anti-inflammatory and anti-bacterial. It is also astringent. It is good on minor skin irritations and burns. To use, dot lavender essential oil onto blemishes individually using a cotton swab. Used once or twice per day on mild acne, this will help dry up the blemishes.

Burdock - Burdock is often taken internally as a tea. The leaves, roots and stems of the burdock plant are rich in minerals that promote sweating and urination (a natural diuretic). For the treatment of acne, use burdock topically, as a face wash. Apply cooled tea to the skin with a washcloth and rinse with cool water.

Calendula - Used as a remedy for many skin ailments, calendula has antibacterial and calming properties. Calendula is often found as a tea. To use, make the tea and allow cooling. Then apply to the face with a cotton ball or cloth. There are also calendula creams available that can be found at your local natural food store. These creams are usually too thick in consistency to help with acne, however, they can be used lightly.

Chamomile - This flowering herb is often found in teas. It contains a natural anti-inflammatory called azulene. Chamomile is used as a skin wash in the treatment of acne. To use, steep chamomile tea and allow cooling. Apply to the skin with a cotton ball or washcloth. You can also dab the mixture onto blemishes. There are also skin care products available with chamomile.

Rose - Rose essential oil has soothing antiseptic properties. It also smells wonderfully. Find rosewater that is made from essential oil. Put some into a spray bottle and spritz onto the face whenever you want.

Grapefruit Seed Extract - The seeds of grapefruit have been found to have potent micro bacterial properties. Mix 5 drops of extract with ½ cup water to dilute and use as a face wash.

Aloe - Aloe has long been known to be a soothing anti-inflammatory with anti-bacterial properties. Use in the gel form for best affects. Use topically by applying directly to the blemish spots.

Altitude Sickness

If you are unaccustomed to higher altitudes, you may have feelings of sickness. These symptoms can range from mild to severe and may feel like a cold or flu. You may get a headache, nausea, weakness and may have trouble sleeping. A headache is the most common complaint associated with altitude sickness. At higher altitudes the amount of oxygen mixed into the air is less. This drop of oxygen can affect the heart, muscles, lungs and nervous system. It can affect anyone, even those in good physical condition. After one to five days the body will begin to adjust and altitude sickness will subside.

The best way to avoid altitude sickness is to ascend slowly. You should also drink plenty of water and avoid drinking alcohol, because this can add to your symptoms. There are some herbs you can take to help prevent altitude sickness as well as lessen the effects on your body. Begin taking these herbs from one to three days before you leave for the higher altitude.

Ginkgo - Ginkgo helps improve circulation and therefore helps improve the body's tolerance to low levels of oxygen. Scientific studies have confirmed these results in humans. Take 120 to 150 milligrams daily. These are usually in the form of capsules. Although not common, side effects are possible. These include headaches and upset stomach.

Reishi - This is an ancient Chinese remedy that helps to improve oxygenation to the blood. Take up to 1,000 milligrams in capsule form each day or two teaspoons of tincture three times per day. Herbalists suggest you take the dosage while at a higher elevation and continue taking it for several days after.

Ginseng - Ginseng has been shown to help improve blood oxygenation and respiratory function. It is also used in treating asthma and bronchitis. Take up to four 500-milligram capsules daily while symptoms persist. Do not combine ginseng with caffeine, antidepressants or blood thinners, and do not use if you are pregnant or have high blood pressure.

Siberian Ginseng - Well known as a tonic herb, Siberian ginseng helps improve overall health when taken long-term. Begin taking a few days before ascending for maximum effect. Take up to nine 500 milligram capsules per day or up to 20 drops of tincture up to three times per day.

Ginger - Ginger is an old cure used for nausea. It can be used for altitude sickness as well as motion sickness. It comes in various forms such as tea, tincture, capsules or raw. Take up to eight 500 milligram capsules daily or ½ to 1 teaspoon of ground root per day or 10 to 20 drops of tincture per day. Dilute tincture in water to drink. Do not take ginger if you have gallbladder disease.

Anxiety

Anxiety is extreme stress, sometimes panic. It can cause symptoms such as shortness of breath along with feelings of doom. You can experience anxiety when your body reacts to signals it thinks are threats. Your heart rate goes up and you start to sweat.

Other causes of anxiety can be classified as phobias, such as fear of flying or fear of heights. Herbs can be an easy way to help ease anxiety naturally. If you are taking anti-depressant drugs, however, do not try to substitute herbal remedies. Talk to your doctor before taking herbal remedies.

When treating anxiety, start with the mildest remedy in the mildest dosage and go from there. Many of the herbs used to treat anxiety are safely compatible.

Oats - Oat seeds are calming and soothing and are helpful for those suffering from daily stress or who feels frayed. Tea is the common method of taking oats. Steep 1 to 2 tablespoons of seeds in a cup of hot water for ten minutes. You can drink a cup of tea every two hours as needed. Tincture is also available and you can take up to 3 teaspoons every two hours. Oats are also available as capsules.

Chamomile - Used often as tea, chamomile has a very soothing and calming effect on you. It helps relax the muscles and also helps ease a tense stomach. Drink one cup of tea every two hours or up to 3 teaspoons of tincture every two hours. Chamomile is readily available as tea at most supermarkets, but it's a good idea to keep some on hand.

Linden - Linden gently relaxes and eases muscle tension, and is also used as a remedy for high blood pressure. Linden also makes a good all-around remedy for helping keep the cardiovascular system functioning well. It is most often used in tea, and you should drink one cup of tea every two hours as needed. Tincture is also available as well as capsules.

Vervain - Vervain is an herb that soothes and calms the nervous system as well as helps with depression. Often found as a tea, drink one cup of tea every two hours. It is also available as a tincture and in capsules.

Motherwort - This old-time remedy is useful for the cardiovascular system in general. It can help calm nerves and aids in soothing anxiety that can cause a rapid heart rate. Drink one cup of Motherwort tea every two hours. It is also available as a tincture and as capsules. Consult your doctor before taking Motherwort if you are currently taking any cardiac drugs.

Lavender - Lavender is relaxing and uplifting. It is fragrant and offers relief for anxiety and depression. Lavender essential oil is used diluted in bath water or can be inhaled. To use in a bath, add 10 to 12 drops to a full tub. You can also dilute it with oil to use as massage oil. It should not be taken internally.

St. John's Wort - Commonly used to treat depression, St. John's Wort is an overall health booster that helps the nervous system. As a tonic, take up to 3 teaspoons every two hours. It is also available in capsule form.

Skullcap - Used for anxiety and hormonal mood swings, skullcap is relaxing to the nervous system. It can be taken as a tea, a tincture or in capsule form. To make tea, steep one or two teaspoons of dried herbs in a cup of hot water for 10 minutes. Drink one cup of hot tea every two hours as needed.

Kava-Kava - This is an anti-anxiety herb that originated in the South Pacific islands. It works similarly to Valium, working with the part of the brain that controls the nervous system and emotions. It does not cause addiction nor does the body build up a tolerance to it. It also doesn't impair thinking the way drugs may. In fact, in studies it was shown to improve brain function and memory. It is a good solution to treat anxiety on a short-term basis. The standard form is in capsules. Do not take with alcohol.

Valerian - Valerian is considered a strong anti-anxiety herb. Similar to Valium, it works with the central nervous system; however it does not cause dependence. It is also used to improve sleep as well as a muscle relaxant. It is taken in capsule form. Note – a small percentage of users indicate an increase in anxiety when taking this herb. If that happens, discontinue use.

Passionflower - Passionflower is a strong herb used primarily for calming and treating insomnia. It can also be used to help calm daytime anxiety. It is most commonly used as a tea. To make the tea, steep one to two teaspoons of dried herbs in a cup of hot water for 10 minutes. Drink one cup every two hours.

Siberian Ginseng - This herb helps restore adrenal glands that are overstressed. It is a good choice for those who are chronically overstressed, and is taken as a tonic. It has a cumulative effect, meaning that it may take several weeks or even months to see results from taking the tonic.

Arthritis

Arthritis affects more than 40 million Americans of all ages. It is the stiffening or inflammation of the joints, and can occur in any joint, but it commonly starts in the hips, fingers and knees. There are two main types of arthritis, with osteoarthritis being the most common form. It is simply the breaking down or wearing down of the joints with age and worsens over time. Rheumatoid arthritis is a form of an autoimmune disease that causes inflammation and distortion of the joints. There is no cure for arthritis, and doctors prescribe medication to help keep inflammation and pain down.

Herbal remedies include both internal and external mixtures.

Cayenne - Cayenne and other peppers contain analgesics and anti-inflammatory agents called capsaicin. This is often used in creams and other topical mixtures to help relieve pain. Creams come in different strengths.

Evening Primrose - Taken internally, Evening Primrose helps combat inflammation. It can also help with the pain associated in particular with rheumatoid arthritis. Taken in capsule form, take up to 12 capsules per day. It can also be taken as oil, and you should take only ½ teaspoon of oil per day. Be aware that this oil can be expensive.

Green Tea - Green tea has compounds that help the symptoms of rheumatoid arthritis. You'll find green tea products widely available now, and you may drink several cups of green tea per day, and black tea is also beneficial

Yucca - Native Americans have used Yucca for centuries as food and as a remedy, and recent studies have confirmed its effectiveness as a remedy for arthritis. Yucca reduces the swelling and pain of arthritis as well as helps prevent stiffness in the joints. It can be applied topically to affected joints, and can also be taken internally. Capsules are available and you may take up to four 490-milligram capsules per day.

Turmeric - Turmeric is a common Indian spice that is helpful in the treatment of arthritis, because it has anti-inflammatory properties. It can be ingested as well as used topically on affected areas. You can take 250 - 300 milligram capsules up to three times per day or up to one teaspoon per day in food. It is also available as a tincture.

Asthma

Asthma affects about 14 million Americans, many of them children. Asthma is a respiratory disorder triggered by certain allergens, and asthma attacks can come on suddenly and become very severe quickly. People with Asthma need to work closely with their doctor to find suitable remedies. The herbal remedies suggested here have been shown to help.

Ginkgo - This ancient Chinese herb has long been used to help treat asthma, and studies have shown this to be particularly effective against exercise-induced asthma. Treatments require continued use for six to eight weeks at a time for maximum effectiveness. There have been rare cases of skin rash and upset stomach associated with the use of ginkgo. Check with your doctor if you are taking any blood thinners.

Garlic and Onion - Garlic and onion have long been used to treat bronchitis and asthma, and they have been shown to inhibit allergen-induced responses. The ingredient that possesses these characteristics is called quercetin. It can be found as a dietary supplement in health food stores. Allicin, the ingredient in garlic, is available in capsule form as well.

Licorice - This herb has anti-inflammatory properties as well as expectorant and anti-viral properties. It also has been known to stimulate the immune system, a huge factor in the treatment of asthma. Use products from the whole root, rather than the DGL form, which does not contain the active ingredient glycyrrhizin, which is necessary to get the effects desired. Do not take for longer than 6 weeks at a time. Also, do not take if you are pregnant, have high blood pressure or diabetes.

Turmeric - Turmeric is one of the main spices in curry. It contains curcumin, which is known to work as an anti-inflammatory, anti-viral and anti-oxidant. You can easily add turmeric to your spice rack and use it when cooking. It is also available in capsule form and as a tincture. Do not take if you have gallstones.

Ephedra - Ephedra has been known to help with asthma, however, it is no longer a recommended remedy due to possible side effects. Consult with your doctor before taking this herbal remedy.

Bladder Infections

Nearly half of all women suffer from a bladder infection at some time in their life. They are most common in sexually active and pregnant women. Bladder infections can become serious, so if it persists you need to see a doctor as the infection can travel to the kidneys where it can cause more serious damage.

Cranberry - Yes, the old wives tale is actually true. Cranberry juice can help prevent and cure bladed infections by acidifying the urine. In order to be effective, though, you need to drink at least 5 cups of cranberry juice per day. You can also get cranberry in capsule form, which is easier to take. To prevent infections, drink 1-½ cups of unsweetened cranberry juice per day.

Goldenrod - This herb is popular in Europe for treating bladder infections. It is one of the safest and most effective herbs for increasing urine flow and inhibiting bacteria growth. It also helps decrease inflammation. Taken as a tea, drink 2 to 3 cups of tea daily.

Oregon Graperoot - The active ingredient berberine can help kill many types of bacteria that are harmful. It also helps prevent bacteria from sticking to the bladder wall, thus preventing bladder infections. Available as a tincture, take one teaspoon three times per day as needed. Do not use if you are pregnant.

Echinacea - This acts as an anti-bacterial as well as an anti-inflammatory. It also is known to help pump up the immune system, which helps those with frequent bladder infections. If you have an allergy to ragweed, do not take this herb, as you could experience an allergic reaction.

Blisters

The body creates a blister to form a protective pocket of fluid to help heal certain wounds, such as burns and those caused by repeated rubbing. Whenever possible, leave the blister alone to heal. Once a blister pops, however, you need to help keep the new skin clean and free from bacteria. Herbal remedies for blisters are topical.

Calendula - This herb helps heal and has antiseptic and anti-inflammatory properties. It is often found as the main ingredient in crèmes or salves. Calendula is considered a safe herb.

Comfrey - Comfrey is high in allantoin, which stimulates and promotes new skin cell growth. It is available in many prepared crèmes and salves and is considered safe.

Lavender - Lavender helps to speed the healing process, and is also an antiseptic. The scent of lavender is very soothing as well. Lavender is a main ingredient in many lotions and crèmes, and is also available as an essential oil. To use the essential oil, first dilute with water, dampen a clean cloth with the mixture and apply to the blister for several minutes at a time.

St-John's-Wort - Used topically, St-John's Wort has anti-inflammatory and antiseptic properties. Use a clean swab and gently dab the blister with the solution.

Bronchitis

Bronchitis is an inflammation in the bronchi, the passageways from the lungs. It is characterized by a cough that starts dry and progresses to a mucus cough. Bronchitis can be acute or chronic. Acute bronchitis is usually the result of a cold and viral infection. Chronic bronchitis is a persistent cough that lasts more than 3 months, with air pollution and smoking contributing to chronic bronchitis. Herbal remedies can help with both types. If you are having severe symptoms such as chest pain, high fever or are coughing up blood you need to see a medical specialist immediately.

Licorice - Licorice soothes mucous membranes and is an expectorant. It also helps stimulate the cells to produce more interferon, the body's own antivirus. Taken as capsules or as a tincture or tea, licorice should not be taken for longer than 6 weeks.

Horehound - Horehound is available in syrups and also in lozenges. It soothes a sore throat and also works as an expectorant. It is also commonly available as a tea.

Peppermint - Peppermint has menthol properties that help relax airways and also helps fight viruses. It is a good thing to use as an herbal steam. Add 3 to 5 drops of peppermint essential oil to 4 cups of very hot water. Then use a towel to cover your head and tent the steam. Inhale this way until the water stops steaming.

Mullein - A tea or tincture, mullein is used to help you expel mucus. It can also help stop the pain of a raspy cough. Drink up to 6 cups of tea per day.

Wild Cherry Bark - Wild cherry bark is often mixed with other herbs. It helps to suppress coughs, and should only be used for short periods of time. It is best used on coughs that are the dry, hacking type. It is available in teas and tinctures.

Bruises

Most bruises are minor and are easily treated with herbal methods. Herbs can help reduce the swelling associated with the bruise as well as provide pain relief.

Arnica - Arnica is known for its pain relieving properties as well as its antiseptic and anti-inflammatory properties. It can help speed up the healing of a bruise. It is most often used topically, and you can find it as a main ingredient in many herbal salves and ointments. You can also make your own compress using dried arnica flowers. First, steep the dried arnica in hot water for ten minutes. Strain and cool the mixture, and then soak a clean towel in the mixture and apply it to the bruise for about half an hour. Repeat three times per day.

Calendula - Used as a topical anti-inflammatory, calendula also works as an astringent and is antiseptic. It can be applied to a bruise as a cream, gel, salve or compress. To use the dried herb, take the dried flowers and steep them in hot water for 10 minutes. Allow the water to cool and use as a compress on the bruise with a clean towel.

Comfrey - Comfrey contains allantoin, which helps renew skin cells. It is used topically. It is also considered an anti-inflammatory, and is often an ingredient in herbal creams and salves. You may make a compress by steeping the dry herbs in hot water for 10 minutes. Allow to cool, and then soak a clean towel in the mixture and place on the bruise. Keep the compress on for an hour at a time. You may repeat as often as needed.

St.-John's-Wort - This is used as an inflammatory and is used topically to speed the healing process. As oil, it can be applied as needed. You may also find it as an ingredient in some crèmes or salves. Do not use St.-John's-Wort if you are going out in the sun as skin reactions can occur when exposed to sunlight.

Burns

Burns of many kinds are common, and occur to all age groups. They can range from minor to major and are given categories based on severity. First-degree burns affect only the outmost layers of skin. Second-degree burns extend deeper into the skin and produce more redness and swelling as well as blisters. Third-degree burns are the most severe and often require skin grafts. First and second-degree burns can be treated quite easily with topical herbal remedies. Always see a doctor for severe burns or burns that cover areas of your body larger than your hand.

Aloe - Aloe is a common burn aid and is found in many over the counter products. It not only helps soothe the pain but also fights bacteria and reduces inflammation. Find aloe in the gel form if possible and look for products that contain 100% aloe, as they work the best. If you have an aloe plant you can actually use that as well. Cut a piece off one of the "arms" and place the gel-like inner substance right onto the burn area. Aloe works well on sunburns as well as other minor burns.

Calendula - Calendula helps as an anti-inflammatory as well as an antiseptic, and helps in the healing process. Calendula can be found in many over the counter products. For use on burns, find a product that is not too thick. You want the skin to be able to breathe through it.

Comfrey - The active ingredient allantoin helps tremendously in speeding up the healing process of burns. Commercial products are available but you can also use a tea-soaked cloth placed on the burn. To use tea, first steep the tea in hot water for 10 minutes and allow to cool. Then, soak a clean cloth or towel in the mixture and apply to the burned area for a half-hour at a time.

Gotu Kola - A compound in gotu kola helps to stimulate collagen growth to help repair skin. It helps heal burns and all types of wounds and helps keep scarring to a minimum. Apply topically by mixing the powder from capsules with aloe and then applying to the burn area.

Bursitis or Tendonitis

Overuse and misuse of two parts of the joint structures, the bursa and the tendons, can result in long-term inflammation and irritation. Bursitis is likely to occur in the shoulders, elbows, hips and knees while tendonitis affects shoulders, wrists, elbows and knees. It causes pain and often inflammation.

Turmeric - Turmeric is an anti-inflammatory and antioxidant. The active ingredient, curcumin, is responsible for these properties and in studies has shown to be as effective as potent anti-inflammatory drugs, but without the side effects. Turmeric can be taken internally as well as used topically. Take up to 600 milligrams daily. Taken in larger amounts, it can cause stomach irritation.

Cayenne - Used topically or in capsule form, cayenne helps reduce pain naturally. Taken internally, cayenne acts as an antioxidant. Used topically, it will ease the pain and gently improves circulation to the area, making the area warm. When using topically, be sure to wash your hands before touching your eyes or nose.

Licorice - This root helps stop inflammation when taken internally by inhibiting an enzyme in the body. Take a 500-milligram capsule up to three times per day. Licorice is also available as a tincture and tea. Do not take licorice for more than 6 weeks at a time. Do not take if you are pregnant, if you have high blood pressure, diabetes or heart disease.

Devil's Claw - This can reduce pain and swelling and is popular in Europe. The root of this plant is used to make capsules or tincture. Do not take if you have ulcers.

Ginger - Ginger is known to inhibit inflammation and reduce pain. It also has antioxidant properties. Take as a capsule or tincture. It can also be used fresh; eat 1/3 ounce of fresh ginger each day.

Canker Sores

Also known as mouth ulcers, these sores can be painful. They are often associated with food allergies, immune system dysfunction and nutritional deficiencies. If you have them often, talk to your doctor to help determine the cause. Vitamin B12 and folic acid deficiencies can contribute to the cause of canker sores.

Chamomile - a study has shown that chamomile mouthwash is an effective treatment for mouth sores. It helps keep inflammation down and helps promote healing. Drink up to 4 cups of tea per day or cool and use as a mouthwash. You can also make a mouthwash using 10 drops of tincture mixed with water.

Echinacea - Echinacea tincture produces a numbing effect that is helpful in managing the pain associated with canker sores. If the canker sore is large or deep avoid using tinctures as they may cause stinging. Instead, use less concentrated mixtures such as tea.

Gotu Kola - Gotu Kola is used to help promote healing. It has long been known to speed the healing of wounds. It can be taken internally as a hot tea or cold as an oral rinse.

Goldenseal - Goldenseal has antiseptic and anti-inflammatory properties and can help to fight the infection associated with a canker sore. It also can help lessen the pain. Dissolve several drops of tincture in a glass of water and use as a mouth rinse.

Ginkgo - When applied topically, this herb helps promote healing. It is rich in anti-oxidants and is also an anti-inflammatory. Make a tea and use the mixture to swab the sore with a cotton swab.

Carpal Tunnel Syndrome

Carpal Tunnel Syndrome is a disorder that affects many thousands of people each year. It is a compression of a nerve in the wrist often brought on by repeated movements of the wrist and hand, such as keyboarding. Depending on the severity of the disorder, herbal remedies may help with inflammation and blood flow.

Turmeric - A common kitchen spice, turmeric is known to help stop inflammation. Available in capsule form, take one 300-milligram capsule up to three times per day. It is also available as a tincture. The easiest way to get it, however, is to use it as a spice, added to foods. Add 1 teaspoon of spice per day to food.

Boswellia - Boswellia is a tree resin that has been found to help block the chemicals in the body that favor inflammation. Available in capsule form, look for products that contain at least 65 percent boswellia acid in order to be effective.

Ginkgo - Ginkgo is known to help increase blood flow and reduce swelling. It also protects nerves and can help them heal. In capsule form the typical dosage is up to 180 milligrams per day.

Cataracts

Cataracts are a cloudy film that covers the eyes causing vision problems. While usually associated with old age, anyone can get cataracts. They are thought to be caused by overexposure to the sun or diabetes. Outpatient surgery is now a standard procedure and the only way to actually remove cataracts once they have formed. There are some herbs, however, that are helpful in improving vision and eye function.

Bilberry - These berries are thought to improve vision and protect the eyes from disease. The fruits of the bilberry contain antioxidant ingredients that can help prevent clouding of the eyes. Used in capsule form, take up to three capsules per day.

Rosemary - A common herb used in cooking, rosemary contains powerful antioxidants that may help retard the growth of cataracts. Take rosemary as a tea, mixing with lemon balm. Drink at least one cup of hot tea per day.

Turmeric - Turmeric has a high concentration of antioxidants, especially the top three known to help prevent cataracts, vitamins A, C and E. Take up to three 500-milligram capsules per day or use a tincture.

Chronic Fatigue Syndrome

CFS is a debilitating exhaustion that affects thousands of people every year. The illness begins with flu-like symptoms but does not go away. It can progress to cause headaches, depression and anxiety. If you have severe feelings of fatigue it's worth getting checked out by a doctor. Some herbal remedies can be very effective in treating many of the symptoms of CFS.

Astragalus - Often used in Chinese medicine, astragalus is used as an overall tonic to help boost the immune system. It has anti-viral properties, and is safe for long-term use. Available in capsule form, take up to 5 500-milligram capsules per day. It is also available as a tincture.

Echinacea - This popular herb helps improve the immune system. It can be taken as a tea, a tincture or in capsule form. Take for two weeks followed by a one-week break. If you are allergic to daisies beware that this is part of the daisy family.

Reishi - A traditional Chinese remedy, reishi has long been used to help fight inflammations, infections and allergies. It is also a strong anti-oxidant. The most common form is capsule. Take up to three 1,000-milligram capsules two to three times per day.

Siberian ginseng - This helps bolster resistance to stress and increases adrenal function. In studies it has been shown to increase the number of immune cells, helping stave off infections. Taken in capsule form, take up to 4500 milligrams per day.

Cold Sores

Cold sores are small blisters on the lips caused by the herpes simplex virus. They are often brought on by stress, and can last up to 14 days. While oral anti-viral drugs may be prescribed by your doctor to lessen the effects, these have side effects of nausea and headaches. Repeated use of anti-viral drugs can cause viral resistance.

Lemon Balm - Lemon balm is an herb that helps to stop the spread of many viruses, including the herpes simplex virus. Lemon balm is often found as an ingredient in commercial creams. Apply to the affected area up to five times per day as needed. It is also available in capsule form and as a tea to be taken internally.

Licorice - Licorice is a natural anti-inflammatory and in studies has been shown to inactivate the herpes simplex virus. You can apply a licorice compress topically as often as needed. You may also take licorice internally in the form of tea or capsules. Do not use longer than 6 weeks at a time, and do not take if you have heart disease or high blood pressure.

Mullein - The healing properties of this plant helps fight the herpes viruses, and can also soothe irritated skin. You can take it internally, as a tea, or apply topically in a compress.

St.-John's-Wort - St.-John's-Wort contains the compound hypericin, which is known to help fight the herpes virus as well as to help heal wounds. Take 300-milligrams up to three times per day in capsule form. You can also drink tea made from steeping the dried herb. It can also be applied topically by making into a compress. Do not take internally if you are already taking a prescription anti-depressant.

Colds or the Flu

Colds and flu are often viral infections for which there is no cure. There are no drugs that can be taken as a preventative measure against the common cold. While there are many over the counter drugs available to treat the symptoms of colds and flu, you are often just as well off taking herbal remedies, which have fewer side effects.

Echinacea - Studies have shown that this herb can shorten the duration and lessen the severity of a cold. It does this by helping to stimulate the body's own production of anti-viral substances and helps enhance the body's immune cells, helping it better fight off cold germs. (Often available in capsule form, take 900 milligrams of Echinacea per day.)

Astragalus - This Chinese herb has immune-boosting properties, and also has anti-viral properties. Take Astragalus throughout the cold and flu season to help bolster your immune system to avoid getting colds. Commonly found in capsule form, take up to 3600 milligrams per day.

Elderberry - Elderberry has been found to have compounds that help fight the flu. Taken as soon as symptoms start, and continue taking it daily. Commercially available as syrups and lozenges, these can be taken as directed on the package. It is also available as tea, tincture and in capsule form.

Garlic - Garlic helps boost the immune system and fights bacteria and yeast. You can eat garlic in foods, but during cold season it is helpful to take a garlic supplement. It is readily available in capsule form. Take up to 5,000 micrograms per day.

Vitamins - Vitamin C and Zinc are known to help lessen the duration of colds as well as help keep the symptoms down. Take supplements in capsule form or in lozenge form during cold season and especially with the onset of any symptoms.

Constipation

Constipation can happen to you when you have inadequate fluid or fiber intake. Laxatives are available over the counter. You can take an herbal laxative or use herbs to help your problem.

Psyllium seed - These seeds help provide proper fiber in order to keep your system working properly. Available as a powder, it can be added to liquids. Dissolve a tablespoon in an 8-ounce glass of water or juice and drink immediately. Follow with another glass of water. This should be taken daily.

Flaxseed - This is a bulking agent that provides a source of omega-3 essential fatty acids, something lacking in most diets. Mix one teaspoon of ground flaxseed in a glass of water or juice. You can take this up to three times per day.

Cuts and Scrapes

Most cuts and scrapes are minor and do not require a doctor visit. For these minor abrasions, herbs can be used externally in compresses, gels, or salves. The anti-bacterial properties of the herbs will help the cuts heal faster and help keep them from becoming infected.

Calendula - Calendula has long been known to have healing properties. It is often the main ingredient in herbal salves. It promotes the growth of new skin and also helps inhibit bleeding. Used as a cream or salve it is readily available at natural or herbal stores.

Aloe - The soothing properties of aloe make it help with the healing process. It can be used on cuts and scrapes to help promote healing and to aid in pain relief. Aloe can be found in many over the counter brands at your local drug store. Be sure to get gel that has a high percentage of aloe as it works best in its pure state.

Comfrey - Comfrey is a healing herb that is also found in many prepared creams or salves. You can also make a compress by wetting dried comfrey and placing it in a clean cloth. Apply the compress by holding it onto the affected area.

Dandruff

Dandruff is an inflammation of the skin on the head, causing flaking and itching skin on the scalp. Often noticeable, it can be treated with herbal remedies to help keep the flaking to a minimum. Doctors are not sure what causes dandruff but it can flair up during stressful times as well as in the winter when the air is dry.

Evening Primrose - Evening primrose contains an oil that helps rashes as well as dandruff. You can rub the oil into the scalp to help keep the dry skin lubricated. You may also take it in capsule form, typically taking up to 10 capsules per day.

Flaxseed - This has high levels of omega-3 fatty acids which has been known to help with rashes and dandruff. Usually taken internally, take 1 teaspoon per day. You can also rub flaxseed oil directly onto the scalp.

Tea Tree - Known for its anti-fungal properties, tea tree oil is used externally. Add it to evening primrose oil or flaxseed oil and rub the mixture into the scalp before bed. Leave it on overnight, then rinse out in the morning and wash your hair as usual.

Depression

Everyone suffers from some depression from time to time. Depression is a hopeless, sad feeling that doesn't quickly go away. Depression may range from subtle to serious, and the more serious the depression, the more you need to seek medical help. If your depression is not severe, there are some herbal remedies that may help you. Do not take herbal cures while taking prescription medication and do not stop taking your medication unless directed to do so by your doctor.

St.-John's-Wort - This herbal remedy is known for its use to treat depression. Studies have shown that the use of St.-John's-Wort is often as effective as prescription medications and has fewer side effects. You must take this for up to two weeks to start to see the benefits. Take it in capsule form and follow the directions for use, or you can also take it as a tea. It can cause mild stomach upsets or rashes in some people.

Kava-Kava - This herb helps alleviate anxiety that often accompanies depression. It can be taken without the usual side-effects of prescription medication that makes people feel sedated. Taken in capsule form, take up to six 500-milligram capsules per day.

Oats - This plant helps with depression and stress and helps with your overall nervous system. It is the same plant used to make the oatmeal breakfast cereal. Available as a tea, drink up to 3 cups of tea per day.

Diarrhea

Many things, such as virus or bacteria as well as food poisoning can cause diarrhea. Most diarrhea goes away on its own in a matter of a few days. If it lasts longer than a week or is very severe you should see a doctor. There are some herbal remedies that can be very effective in helping treat it.

Agrimony - Agrimony contains an astringent, which has drying properties in the bowel. Available as a tea, steep the dried herbs in hot water for 10 minutes. Then remove the herbs and drink the tea. You may drink up to 3 cups of tea per day as needed.

Blackberry and Raspberry Leaf - Another astringent, the roots of these plants can help relieve diarrhea. Taken as a tea, you can take up to 3 cups of tea per day.

Oregon Graperoot and Goldenseal - These related herbs contain berberine, which has been shown to be effective in treating the bacteria that can cause diarrhea. Available in capsule form, take up to 6 500-milligram capsules per day.

Apples - Apples are a natural source of pectin, which is a very common anti-diarrhea remedy. Pectin is an ingredient in many over the counter remedies that helps add bulk. Eat apples or applesauce, but avoid apple juice as this tends to have the opposite effect.

Diverticulosis

Diverticulosis is small pockets that form in the colon, common in those over the age of 40. These pockets can become inflamed, which in some cases can become infected. There are some herbal remedies that can be taken as a preventative to help keep the colon clear.

Psyllium - Psyllium is found in India and is rich in mucilage, water soluble fiber. The husks of this plant can be ground up and stirred into water, and can also be taken in capsule form. Psyllium is also available in many commercial products. Start with small doses and work your way up to full dosages.

Cat's Claw - Long used in South American folk medicine, cat's claw is safe to use. It helps treat infections, arthritis and intestinal disorders. You can find this herb available in capsule form or as a tincture or tea.

Aloe Vera - Aloe gel has healing properties when applied directly to the skin. It helps relieve burns, and has anti-inflammatory properties. When taken orally as a capsule, take up to 8 capsules per day.

Ear Infections

Ear infections are common in swimmers, thus a common name for one type of ear infection is "swimmer's ear". Ear infections are common in small children because their ear canals and tubes are not large enough to keep fluid from accumulating in them when they have a cold or flu. The accumulated mucus can become infected. Taking herbal cures instead of antibiotics can often help cure the infection. Besides taking herbs to help cure the infection, you can also try making some "swimmer's drops" to put into the ear.

Echinacea - Taken internally, this ancient Chinese herb is known to help treat infections. You may take capsules or a tincture, and is also available as a tea. Note that you may be allergic to this herb if you are allergic to ragweed or other members of the aster family.

Astragalus - Another ancient Chinese remedy that is taken orally, astragalus is helpful in treating infections, and can be taken as a preventative remedy. Available as capsules or in tincture form, this is usually safe for children. For young children, check with the doctor before administering.

Oregon Graperoot - The berberine in Oregon Graperoot acts as a natural antibiotic. It is used to kill many types of bacteria. It is taken internally in capsule form, and you should follow the directions on the bottle. Do not take if you are pregnant.

Lemon Balm - A good-tasting herb, lemon balm is a natural anti-virus, bacteria fighting herb and is also used to help calm or soothe. Commonly available as a tea, drink up to 4 cups of tea per day.

Eczema

Eczema is a dry skin condition that affects many adults and children. It occurs in patches that can become thick and red, and it can often occur in those with allergies such as hay fever. Topical creams can be applied to help the skin recover. Herbal remedies do not have the side effects that some prescriptions can have.

Licorice - The anti-inflammatory properties of licorice helps calm the skin when eczema flares up. It acts much like cortisol but without the side effects. It can be taken internally as a tea or externally by making a compress of the steeped herbs.

Burdock - Known to decrease inflammation, burdock is a traditional herb, which has been used for years to help skin disorders. Besides helping inflammation, it also contains insulin that helps the body fight off skin bacteria. Taken as a tea; drink up to 4 cups per day. It can also be used topically. Simmer the dried root in hot water for 10 minutes. Strain and apply the cooled liquid to the affected skin area.

Echinacea - Echinacea is an American wildflower that has substances that can help fight infection as well as decrease inflammation. It can be found as a main ingredient in many prepared herbal skin crèmes.

Comfrey - Comfrey contains allantoin, an ingredient in many skin lotions. It soothes the skin and helps speed up healing. Apply as a salve or lotion. Do not use if pregnant.

Eyestrain

Eyestrain can occur in those who overuse their eyes, or can be caused by other factors such as tension or anxiety. Eyestrain is characterized by headaches, blurry vision or difficulty focusing. If you have mild eyestrain every so often it is not a cause for alarm. Some herbal remedies can be helpful.

Eyebright - This herb helps reduce watery eyes as it has both anti-inflammatory and astringent properties. It also helps relieve eye irritation. Most often taken as a tea, drink 1 to 3 cups per day. It can also be used as a compress. Steep the dried herbs in hot water for 10 minutes. Strain and cool the liquid then soak a clean towel and apply to closed eyes.

Bilberry - This shrub produces berries that are used to treat vision problems. It helps strengthen the capillaries of the eyes. Taken in capsule form; take 2 to 3 capsules per day. The closely related cranberry, blueberry and huckleberry are also good for treating eye problems.

Goldenseal - Use goldenseal as a compress on the eyes. It contains berberine, which is known to help constrict the blood vessels, helping to get rid of bloodshot eyes.

Fatigue

Everyone feels fatigued from time to time. If you feel fatigue every day for long periods of time, you should consult with a physician, as this may be an underlying symptom of something else. If, however, you experience fatigue occasionally there are some herbal treatments that will help.

Siberian Ginseng - The properties of this herb help improve mental function. It also is thought to aid in the treatment of viral infections. Taken daily, this herb is safe for long-term use. Take in capsule form and follow the specific directions.

Chinese Ginseng - Similar to Siberian Ginseng, Chinese Ginseng has long been used in traditional Chinese medicine. Some forms of this herb can be very strong so it is suggested that you start with low dosages of capsules and work up to larger doses if needed. Do not take if you have high blood pressure or are pregnant.

Licorice - Licorice increases energy and has anti-inflammatory properties, and is known to help the adrenal glands. Taken as a tea, do not take for longer than six weeks.

Astragalus - This traditional herb is used as an energy tonic. It is thought to strengthen the immune system and helps aid digestion. Drink up to 3 cups of tea per day or take in capsule form.

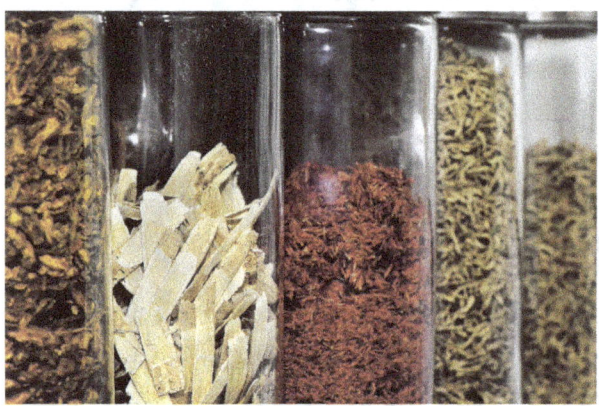

HERBAL REMEDIES G-L

Gas

Gas or flatulence occurs in everyone. If your gas is severe it can become uncomfortable and painful. Certain foods are known to produce gas, and you can avoid these foods if gas is a problem for you. These foods are broccoli, potatoes, dairy products and beans. Swallowing too much air while eating can also produce gas. There are some herbal remedies that can help treat gas.

Peppermint - Peppermint contains menthol, which helps stimulate the intestines. It also helps relax the muscles in the digestive tract, promoting burping. You can eat peppermint candy or mints, which are helpful (Do you always notice the peppermint candies at restaurants?) Peppermint tea is also a great way to take peppermint. You can drink 1–2 cups of tea after a meal to aid digestion.

Chamomile - Chamomile helps aid digestion and can also help dissipate gas in the body. It is also used as an anti-inflammatory. Often used as a tea, it is helpful to drink a cup of chamomile tea after eating. Those with allergies to ragweed should avoid this herb.

Aniseed - The seeds from the anise plant have been shown to help eliminate gas buildup. Taken as a tea; steep the dried, crushed seeds in hot water for 10 minutes. Strain and drink warm.

Ginger - Ginger root is known to help relieve nausea and helps with simple indigestion such as gas. You can drink a cup of tea after a meal that may cause gas. It is also available in capsule form.

Gum Disease

Gum disease is common in adults. Approximately 3 out of 4 adults have some stage of gum disease. It can produce red, swollen or bleeding gums as well as bad breath. Keep your teeth and gums clean to prevent the disease. Herbal remedies that fight bacteria are helpful in keeping the disease in check.

Echinacea - Known for its infection-fighting properties, Echinacea is helpful in reducing bacteria in the mouth that contribute to gum disease. You can use it as a mouth rinse or you can swab it onto swollen gums. It can also be taken in capsule form.

Goldenseal - A compound in the root of this plant is an antibacterial substance. It can help with gingivitis, and is also used to help keep the gums healthy. Taken in capsule form, take up to 6 500-milligram capsules per day. Do not use if you have heart problems or are pregnant.

Calendula - With its beneficial healing properties, calendula is helpful as an anti-viral and anti-inflammatory. It also helps with sore throats. For use on the gums, apply calendula tincture directly to the affected area several times per day.

Aloe - Aloe has soothing properties on skin and gums. You can find aloe as an ingredient in some mouth rinses. You can also swab some aloe onto sore gums as needed; however, you should not swallow aloe gel.

Hangovers

Most adults have had at least one experience with drinking too much alcohol and ending up with a hangover. It can cause a headache, fatigue, nausea and dizziness. To prevent a hangover, do not drink to excess. However, if you do imbibe too much you can help a hangover with herbal remedies.

Willow - There are pain-relieving ingredients in the bark of the willow, and you should take this remedy as a tea. To make the tea, steep willow bark in hot water for 10 minutes, strain and drink.

Dandelion - Dandelion is known to stimulate the liver, which may help in alcohol dissipation. It is also a source of anti-oxidants and can help with stomachaches.

Ginkgo - Gingko helps improve circulation and helps relieve dizziness. For these reasons it may be a good hangover remedy.

Honey and Fruit - The fructose in fruit and honey helps speed up the metabolism of alcohol and helps to decrease the effects of a hangover. If you just can't think about eating a piece of fruit, have a cup of warm tea with honey.

Hay Fever and Allergies

Hay fever is an allergy to certain weeds and flowers that occurs most often in spring and summer. Allergies occur year-round. People can be allergic to many things, but the most common allergies are to pet dander and pollen. Herbal remedies are most effective for those with mild forms of allergies. If you are currently taking prescription medication for allergies consult your doctor before taking herbal remedies.

Stinging Nettle - Studies have found that this herb works as well as conventional medications for treating the symptoms of hay fever. Stinging nettle is available in capsule form.

Peppermint - The anti-inflammatory properties of peppermint help to calm mucous membranes. The scent of peppermint when inhaled helps you feel as though you can breathe easier. You may drink tea or you can steep the peppermint and breathe in the steam.

Licorice Root - The anti-allergy properties of licorice act similarly to cortisone drugs but without the side effects. For hay fever be sure to get whole licorice, not the type labeled DGL, which is used for ulcers.

Garlic - Garlic contains an anti-inflammatory substance called quercetin, which can help calm an allergic response in the body.

Headaches

Headaches occur in everyone from time to time. They are commonly a dull ache that happens in the temple or forehead and comes on during the day. Migraine headaches are a result of insufficient blood flow to the brain, and should be treated by a doctor to determine any underlying cause. Herbal remedies can be helpful in treating regular headaches, and be sure to drink water when you have a headache. Many low-grade headaches are actually caused by a mild form of dehydration.

Feverfew - Feverfew contains substances that inhibit the release of mood hormones in the brain. For best results, use fresh feverfew. When that isn't available, take as a tea or in capsule form.

Bay - There have been some doctors who recommend taking feverfew with bay to prevent a migraine headache. You can often find a combination available in a health food store.

Ginger - Ginger has long been known to relieve and also to prevent headaches. It is an anti-inflammatory and also has substances that help reduce pain. Take in capsule form, according to directions.

Peppermint - Taken internally or used externally, peppermint can help relieve a headache. To take internally, drink peppermint tea. To use externally, mix several drops of peppermint oil with lotion or body oil and massage into the temples.

Heartburn

Heartburn is a pain that occurs in the chest after eating. It is caused by stomach acid that gets into the esophagus causing a painful burning sensation. Symptoms can range from mild to severe. There are many over the counter remedies that can help, but there are also some herbal cures to help the situation.

Licorice Root - This herb can help speed up the healing process in the digestive tract. It is also soothing to the mucous membranes. Look for the type called DGL, as this is better for digestive disorders. Take licorice in capsule form or as a mild tea, which can be taken after a meal.

Aloe Juice - Aloe juice has a calming effect on the digestive tract and may be helpful in the treatment of heartburn. Make your own aloe remedy by mixing powdered aloe with water.

Cabbage Juice - The active ingredient in cabbage can actually help heal ulcers by helping them repair themselves. Drink a cup of the juice after meals.

Calendula - Calendula is used for many types of minor cuts and abrasions and is safe to use. Drink as a tea. To make the tea, steep 2 teaspoons of the dried flowers in hot water for 10 minutes. Strain and drink warm.

Hemorrhoids

Hemorrhoids are painful swollen and inflamed tissues near the rectum, and they may burn and itch. Herbal remedies can actually help strengthen the blood vessels and reduce inflammation associated with hemorrhoids.

Ginkgo - This helps strengthen the blood vessels and also has anti-inflammatory properties. Taken internally, it can be used as a tea, tincture or in capsule form.

Horse Chestnut - This has long been used as an anti-inflammatory, as it helps to decrease swelling. It is also astringent, which helps lessen bleeding. You can use this herb topically in a cream or internally as a tea or in capsule form. To use externally you can use strong-brewed tea to soak the affected area.

Witch Hazel - Witch hazel is a common remedy that is available at the drug store. Apply topically to the affected area, and do not take internally.

Dandelion - Dandelion roots have laxative properties that help with constipation that often accompanies hemorrhoids. To make a tea, steep dried, chopped root for 10 minutes in hot water. Strain and drink warm.

High blood pressure is common in many adults. A number of factors can contribute to high blood pressure, including genetics, and can be aggravated by being overweight. If you are currently taking prescription medication for high blood pressure, do not take herbal cures or stop your current treatment until you discuss this with your doctor.

Hawthorn - The leaves, flowers and berries are used to make tonic that helps improve the cardiovascular system. It helps reduce blood pressure by relaxing the walls of the arteries. This herb takes weeks or months to show any affects so do not rely on this as your sole method of controlling your high blood pressure.

Reishi - This mushroom is known for its rejuvenating properties and has been used since ancient times in Japan and China. It can help reduce your cholesterol. The most common way to take this is in capsule form but it is also available as a powder that can be mixed into liquids.

Garlic - Garlic has been used to cure many ailments for thousands of years, and it is known to help lower blood pressure and cholesterol. You can eat raw or lightly cooked garlic every day. If you prefer, you can take garlic in capsule form, which is readily available.

Dandelion - Dandelion helps increase urine flow and lowers blood pressure. You can eat the leaves in a salad or drink tea. It is also available in capsule form.

High Cholesterol

High cholesterol is very common in adults, and can lead to heart disease, strokes and other serious health problems. You should have your cholesterol level checked by a doctor every year. The levels will indicate if you need to take action to lower your cholesterol. Herbal remedies can be very helpful in lowering cholesterol, but do not substitute herbal remedies for prescription medication. If you are currently under a doctor's care for high cholesterol, check with him before making any changes.

Guggul - An ancient Indian medicine, guggul is known to help lower cholesterol and triglycerides while increasing the HDL, or good cholesterol. Take 25-milligrams three times per day, with meals. It will take up to several months to see any results from taking this supplement.

Artichoke - A substance in artichoke, cynarin, is known to help the body block absorption of cholesterol. It also assists the liver in breaking down toxins. Take up to 3,000-milligrams per day with meals.

Garlic - Long known for its medicinal powers, garlic is helpful in inhibiting the production of cholesterol in the body.

Hives

Hives are itchy red skin patches of irritated skin that is raised and bumpy. It is considered to be an allergic reaction to foods, medications or insect bites. They can also be caused by mold, pollen and animal dander. Mild cases of hives can successfully be treated with herbal remedies. If your hives are severe or cause you to have breathing problems see a doctor immediately.

Licorice - Licorice has anti-inflammatory and anti-allergy properties that help it act to limit the allergen reaction in the body. For this purpose, use whole licorice. You can chop up the root and use in tea or you can steep in hot water, strain and apply the cooled liquid to the hives.

Chamomile - This herb has anti-inflammatory properties. It is also helpful in falling asleep. Most often used as a tea, drink up to 4 cups per day. It can also be applied to the hives topically.

Burdock - The roots, seeds and leaves of this plant all have medicinal properties to help many types of skin problems. Drink as a tea or take in capsule form following bottle instructions.

Aloe - The gel inside the leaves of this plant are well known for their use in helping minor skin irritations and burns. It is also helpful for hives, as it calms the skin and reduces itching. Commercial aloe products are readily available. Choose a product that is close to 100% aloe for the best benefit.

Indigestion

Indigestion is common and happens to everyone at one time or another. Occasional indigestion can be easily treated with herbal remedies. If your indigestion is frequent or severe it could signal an underlying problem and should be checked out by a doctor.

Chamomile - Well known as a soothing herb, chamomile tea can help dispel gas and relax tense stomach muscles. Taken as tea, drink 3 to 4 cups of hot tea per day. You can also use this as a tincture.

Peppermint - Mint aids in digestion because it acts as a muscle relaxant in the stomach and can help calm the whole digestive tract. To be most effective use the tincture or essential oil mixed into water and drink. If heartburn is your problem, peppermint may aggravate the esophagus.

Marshmallow - This plant is used to soothe the mucous membranes in the digestive tract. The root is the part of the plant that is typically used. Most often used in capsule form, take up to 6 500-milligram capsules per day.

Angelica - Angelica stimulates digestion, calms nerves and can help dispel gas and bloating. It is often included in preparations with other herbs, such as dandelion. This herb may cause sensitivity to the sun.

Insect Bites and Stings

Insect bites are usually harmless but can be annoying and painful. They can cause pain and inflammation to the spot of the bite. Herbal remedies can be helpful in dealing with both the pain and swelling of the insect bite. If you are allergic to insect stings, are stung multiple times or are stung on the neck you should seek medical attention.

Aloe - The soothing properties of aloe help hasten healing. It also has anti-bacterial properties. If you have a live plant simply cut a small piece of leaf and scoop out the gel and apply to the bite. Commercial aloe products are readily available at drug stores.

Witch Hazel - Witch hazel has astringent properties and helps shrink swollen tissue. Apply to the bite with a clean cotton swab. It is a good idea to have this on hand for emergencies.

Calendula - Calendula is an anti-inflammatory, anti-bacterial herb that helps wounds heal. It can be found in many commercial preparations at your local health store. Apply directly to the sting as needed.

Comfrey - A substance called allantoin is found in comfrey, which has antiseptic properties and also promotes healing. You can use fresh, crushed comfrey leaves to apply directly to the bite. It is also available in many salves and lotions. Do not ingest.

Insomnia

Insomnia affects millions of people - there are times when you just can't get to sleep. Instead of taking prescription medications that can be harmful or addictive, try an herbal cure.

Valerian - This herb is known to help you sleep and does not have any side effects, such as morning grogginess that is associated with prescription medications. It can help improve sleep quality as well. Take in capsule form according to package directions.

Lemon Balm - Most often available as a good tasting tea, this herb not only helps ease insomnia but also calms nerves and fights fevers. It is also good for headaches and helps calm the digestive tract.

Passionflower - This herb has been shown to calm nerves and decrease anxiety. If you suffer from sleeplessness due to an overactive mind, this will help calm it. Take as a tea before bedtime. Do not mix this herb with MAO antidepressants.

Kava-Kava - This herb helps calm and relax muscles and is known to aid the brain in promoting sleep. Take in capsule form according to the instructions. Do not take kava-kava if you are taking sedatives, and do not use while pregnant.

Chamomile - Chamomile is known for its relaxing properties, and is a gentle sleep aid. Most effective in tea form, drink a cup of warm chamomile tea before bed.

Irritable Bowel Syndrome

IBS is a very common ailment that particularly affects women, but can also affect men. The symptoms are constipation and diarrhea with severe bloating and cramping. If your IBS happens infrequently, try these herbal remedies.

Peppermint - Peppermint is helpful in many digestive disorders because it has soothing properties in the digestive tract. It helps stop cramping and is an anti-inflammatory. Use peppermint oil in capsule form to be most effective in treating this problem.

Psyllium - These seeds help aid the intestinal tract whether the problem is constipation or diarrhea. Stir the dried seed husks into a large glass of water or juice and drink immediately. Drink one glass per day to keep IBS at bay.

Chamomile - Chamomile helps calm the stomach and intestinal tract. It helps to stop muscle spasms that sometimes occur with IBS. You can drink as a tea, up to 4 cups per day between meals. It is also commonly available in capsule form. Do not take if you have allergies to ragweed.

HERBAL REMEDIES M-R

Macular Degeneration

Macular degeneration is an eye disease that affects the center of the retina, eventually causing blindness. It may be caused by cell damage that occurs when there are free radicals, and the body cannot produce enough antioxidants to counteract the process. Some herbal supplements have been found to help slow the progression of the disease.

Bilberry - This herb is rich in anthocyanoside and is known for its antioxidant properties. Take in capsule form as directed on the side of the bottle. Side effects from bilberry can include dizziness and headaches in rare instances.

Ginkgo - This is known to have powerful antioxidant properties and can actually improve vision in those with macular degeneration. Take 40 to 60-milligram capsules three times per day.

Memory Loss

Memory loss is common in people over 50, but it can occur in all ages and the memory loss increases with age. It does not occur at a specific rate. Some herbal remedies have been found to help keep memory loss to a minimum.

Ginkgo - Used for centuries in China, this ancient cure helps strengthen memory and improve circulation. Taken daily, it can be found in capsule form as well as extract. Do not take if you are currently taking prescription blood-thinning medication.

Bacopa - Often called the water hyssop, this plant has been used for its medicinal properties since ancient times. It can strengthen the memory and enhances the conductivity of the nerve tissue. It can be found in commercially prepared formulas specifically for memory loss symptoms.

Club Moss - An ancient Chinese medicinal herb, club moss has been found to help treat memory loss and symptoms of dementia. An ingredient, Huperzine A, can be found in many health food stores. It is also used to treat the beginning stages of Alzheimer's disease. Available in capsule form, take up to 1000-micrograms twice a day.

Menopause

All women go through menopause as they age. Some will experience symptoms such as mood swings, hot flashes and night sweats. Because the body is going through hormonal changes it can take years to readjust to the new levels. Some herbal remedies can treat symptoms that are less severe. If you are taking hormone replacement drugs consult with your physician before taking herbal remedies.

Black Cohosh - Useful as both a menopause and a pre-menstrual remedy, this herb helps by mimicking estrogen in the body. It is also helpful in stopping hot flashes and in minimizing depression. Take in capsule form, and do not exceed the recommended dosage on the bottle.

Dang Ghui - Used in ancient Chinese medicine, this herb helps with many symptoms of menopause. It works in much the same way as estrogen replacements work but in a milder way and without the side effects. Taken in capsule form, take up to 6 500-milligram capsules per day. Do not use if pregnant.

Red Raspberry - Red raspberry is known to strengthen the uterus, helps decrease heavy menstrual flow and relaxes muscles. Take as a tea, and drink one or two cups per day.

Licorice Root - Used in ancient Chinese medications for female reproductive problems, this herb helps control water retention and breast tenderness. It also decreases symptoms associated with the fluctuation of hormones such as what occurs in menopause.

Menstrual Problems

Many women feel various symptoms that are associated with their menstrual cycle. These include moodiness, fatigue, cramps and headaches. While over-the-counter medications can help with some of the symptoms, you may want to try some herbal remedies that can help without side effects.

Vitex - This tree berry extract is good for many menstrual symptoms, including fluid retention, moodiness, food cravings, and acne. It helps by regulating the pituitary gland. Take in capsule form. Do not use during pregnancy, and do not use if you are taking oral contraceptives, as vitex may lessen their effectiveness.

Black Cohosh - Also used to help the symptoms associated with menopause, this powerful herb helps relieve cramps, and helps with pain as well. You must take this herb for a few weeks for it to be effective. Most often taken as a tincture; take 3 to 4 droppers twice a day.

Cramp Bark - This herb gets its name from its use as an antispasmodic. It is safe to use and will relax uterine cramping. It can be combined with valerian or kava-kava. Take as a tea or in capsule form. You can find it mixed with other herbs in mixtures designed to treat PMS.

Kava-Kava - A calming herb, kava-kava helps ease anxiety. It also has pain-relieving effects similar to aspirin. It is recommended to start taking this several days before your period and through your period.

Morning Sickness

Many pregnant women experience morning sickness during pregnancy. The exact cause is not known, however it is likely due to hormonal and metabolic changes that are occurring. Some herbs may offer help for morning sickness, but do not take any herbal remedy while pregnant until you discuss it first with your doctor.

Ginger - Ginger helps calm the stomach and can stop nausea and vomiting. It is also a cure for motion sickness, and it can also reduce gas and bloating. The gentlest dosage is to take as a tea.

Chamomile - Chamomile is soothing and gentle on the digestive system. It is best used as a tea to help calm and relieve nausea. You can sip the tea as needed throughout the day whenever you have symptoms of morning sickness.

Peppermint - Soothing to the digestive tract, this gentle herb is safe to use. It can improve symptoms of bloating and gas. Steep a tea by putting 2 teaspoons of dried peppermint leaves into hot water for 10 minutes. Strain and drink the tea warm.

Motion Sickness

Motion sickness is nausea brought on by motion, such as riding in a car or plane. It can affect anyone and can come on without warning. Some herbal cures may help alleviate the nausea and make the stomach feel better.

Ginger - This herb acts to help dispel gas and settle the stomach. Studies have found it to be more effective than Dramamine. It has also been found to reduce vomiting after surgery. It is most effective when taken several hours before your car ride. Often taken in capsule form, it can be taken as a tincture in water, so even children can take it. Candied ginger is also effective.

Peppermint - Peppermint has been found to prevent vomiting and quiets muscle spasms in the stomach. It is found in many common peppermint candies. The tincture can be mixed with water and taken after meals and before trips.

Fennel - Fennel seeds have long been known to aid with digestion and help calm the stomach. You can use this as a flavoring on foods or take as a tincture or tea.

Nausea

Everyone has a bout of nausea from time to time. It can be brought on by the flu, but often there is no real reason for feeling nauseous. If you are sick, make sure you frequently drink small amounts of liquids to stay hydrated. Some herbal cures may help alleviate the symptoms.

Ginger - Ginger is readily available in many forms and is safe to use. It is effective in reducing nausea and helps quiet the stomach. Extremely versatile, it can be taken as a tea, in crystallized form, dried, powdered or as a tincture. It is also available in capsule form.

Peppermint - Peppermint settles the stomach, and you have probably noticed that peppermint candies are often given at restaurants. If you have a headache or a cold, peppermint is also a good choice for these ailments. Keep peppermint lozenges in the car to help tame nausea while driving. It can also be taken as a tea or tincture.

Lemon Balm - Lemon balm helps the body to deal with and expel excess gas. It can also relieve spasms. The flavor is also pleasing. Make a tea by steeping dried herbs in hot water for 10 minutes, then strain and drink.

Chamomile - This herb is useful for all sorts of ailments and acts to calm nausea. Mild enough for children, this herb is a safe choice in treating many illnesses. Use as a tea or put drops of the tincture into water and drink.

Osteoporosis

Osteoporosis affects millions of people, mostly women. It is a gradual loss of bone density, making people more susceptible to broken and fractured bones. Calcium supplements are important to avoid getting Osteoporosis. Some herbal supplements are available to add to the mineral intake.

Stinging Nettle - This is a natural multi-vitamin that contains calcium, iron, magnesium, phosphorus and proteins. Capsules are the best method of taking this herb. Take up to six 500-milligram capsules daily.

Red Clover - This clover contains compounds that act as a mild form of estrogen, and can help with symptoms of menopause. Take up to five 500-milligram capsules daily. It can also be taken as a tea. Drink up to 3 cups of tea per day.

Horsetail - This traditional remedy helps the body to process calcium. It also provides a natural source of silica that helps strengthen hair, nails and bones. This is readily available in capsule form. Take up to six 500-milligram capsules per day.

Parkinson's Disease

Parkinson's disease is a serious progressive disorder that affects the central nervous system. People with this disease increasingly lose their ability to control muscle movements. The exact cause of Parkinson's disease is not known but it is thought that heredity may play a role. Medical evaluation and treatment are necessary, but some herbal remedies may provide some help. Check with your doctor before adding these to your regime.

Ginkgo - The leaves of this ancient Chinese herb help boost brain function by providing more oxygen to the cells. This may help slow the later stages of Parkinson's. Take up to 60-milligram capsules two or three times per day.

Grapeseed - This provides powerful anti-oxidants, called procyanidins, that can help rid the body of toxins. Taken in capsule form; use as directed on the bottle.

Evening Primrose - The oil from this seed is high in GLAs (or gamma-linolenic acids) that have been found to help the brain chemistry. It can sometimes help the shaking that is often associated with Parkinson's disease. Take in capsule form or take 2 teaspoonfuls per day.

Pinkeye and Sties

Also known as conjunctivitis, pinkeye is a highly contagious inflammation of the eyelid membrane, and causes the white of the eye to appear pink. Pinkeye usually clears up within several days. Sties are small pimples or blocked hair follicles on the eyelid, and can be painful. They open and go away in several days. There are some herbal remedies that can be effective in the treatment of both eye conditions.

Eyebright - This herb is effective in helping soothe many eye problems. It has anti-bacterial properties, and should be used as eyewash or in a compress. Soak a clean cloth in the warm liquid and hold on closed eyes.

Green Tea - This helps aid in the reduction of inflammation and fights infections. Use as a compress. Steep the tea for 10 minutes in hot water, and soak a clean towel with the liquid and place on closed eyes. Hold on the eyes for at least 10 minutes.

Herbal Eyewash - Make eyewash using a mixture of herbs. Steep the herbs in piping hot water for ten minutes. Strain the herbs, leaving the warm liquid. Soak a clean washcloth in the liquid, ring out the excess and place on your closed eyes for 10 minutes.

Pneumonia

Pneumonia often starts with a bad cold but spreads to the lungs, where it causes infection. You may have a mucous cough and may have difficulty taking a deep breath. Severe pneumonia often requires a hospital stay. Mild pneumonia may be treated with herbal remedies, especially if you are prone to this type of condition. Always have your condition checked by a doctor to ensure that it does not progress in severity.

Echinacea - This immune boosting herb is often effective by helping the body fight off infections. This is available in capsule form as well as in a tea or tincture.

Goldenseal - This herb helps fight bacteria and can also help stimulate the body's immune system. You can take this in capsule form or as a tea or tincture. In capsule form, take up to 1,000-milligrams three times per day.

Mullein - This herb is known to help the respiratory tract and can help fight inflammation. It also eases coughs, helping the body get needed rest. Usually used as a tea; steep the dried root in hot water for 10 minutes. Remove the herbs and drink the tea. You may drink up to 3 cups of tea per day.

Poison Ivy and Poison Oak

Allergic reactions to poison ivy and poison oak range from mild to severe. Reactions start with red and itching skin followed by blisters and oozing. If exposed, rinse the affected area as soon as possible with water. For severe reactions you should seek medical attention by a doctor. Mild reactions, however, are often easily helped with herbal remedies.

Jewelweed - This plant is known to help skin rashes caused by poison ivy, oak and sumac. Use the fresh, crushed leaves in a compress and hold on the effected skin. You can also apply a tea rinse to the skin. Mix a strong tea and apply to the skin with a clean cloth.

Aloe - The juice from the aloe plant helps heal wounds and acts as an anti-inflammatory. You can use it right off the plant by breaking off a small piece and applying the gel directly to the skin. Aloe lotion is available commercially. Look for gel that is 100% aloe.

Witch Hazel - This herb is cooling, soothing and drying, three things that will help heal rashes quickly. Readily available at drug stores, apply topically to the skin as often as needed. You can soak a cloth with witch hazel and lay over the effected skin area.

Cucumber - Cucumber acts as a coolant and helps calm inflamed skin. You can use a fresh cucumber applied directly to the skin. You may also mash the cucumber and use by placing small amounts on the skin.

Scabies

Scabies are small lesions that are caused by small bed bugs or mites that bite and burrow into the skin. Most often these small bites do not become infected, however, in those with compromised immune systems, the likelihood of infection increases.

Neem - The oil from this tree has anti-fungal and anti-bacterial properties. It is used topically. Apply to the skin on effected areas, and do not take internally.

Tea Tree Oil - This oil helps fight against parasites, a cause of scabies. Mix 1 part tea tree oil with 5 parts vegetable oil and apply to the skin before bedtime. Do not take internally.

Clove - Essential oil of clove has analgesic properties and is an anti-inflammatory. It also helps protect against bacterial infections, which can make scabies worse. Used topically, mix clove oil with vegetable oil and apply to the skin. Use with caution. Apply to a small area first to make sure that it does not irritate the skin.

Tansy - The herb tansy has long been used to keep insects away and works well in protecting against mites. To use, make a strong tea using dried herbs. Strain the liquid and let cool. Apply the cooled wash to the skin before bedtime.

Shingles

Shingles is a disease that comes from the dormant chicken pox virus. It often occurs in older people and those with compromised immune systems. A strong burning pain or tingling often in the torso and arms or legs characterizes the disease.

Cayenne - Cayenne or chili peppers are useful in easing the pain of shingles. These peppers contain capsaicin, which is an ingredient in many topical creams. You can use commercial creams or make your own blend by mixing a small amount of cayenne powder with lotion or aloe. Apply to the affected areas.

Lemon Balm - This lemon scented herb helps the body fight viruses. You can find lemon balm cream sold commercially, and the product is safe for all ages. You can also take lemon balm internally, most commonly as a tea.

Licorice - The licorice has virus-fighting ingredients that can inhibit the herpes simplex virus. It also fights inflammation and can be used instead of products containing cortisone without the side effects. Taken internally, it can be used as a tea and is often blended with other herbs for taste. Do not take for longer than 6 weeks at a time, and do not take licorice if you have high blood pressure or a history of heart disease.

Baikal Skullcap - This is an herb that has been used since ancient times in China. It fights bacteria and infections, so it is helpful in treating shingles as well as many other conditions. Used topically, you can make a paste using the ground root mixed with water. Apply the paste to the affected areas as needed.

Sinus Infections

Sinus infections are infections of the sinus cavities, located in the cheeks, ears and forehead. Often caused by viruses, the infections can be particularly hard to get rid of. A bad cold or hay fever can turn into a sinus infection, and they often happen to people who smoke. They can sometimes effectively be treated with herbal remedies.

Echinacea - This herb helps boost the immune system and is known to help fight off infections, particularly sinus infections. Take as soon as you feel an infection coming on and continue to take every two hours. You need to take it frequently at the onset of the illness in order to get the best results. You can take up to nine 400-milligram capsules per day.

Astragalus - Taken over a long period of time, astragalus helps boost the immune system slowly. It builds up the immune system of people who get sinus infections often, and is most commonly taken in capsule form.

Oregon Graperoot - This herb is an antimicrobial, as well as astringent and an anti-inflammatory. It can be used to treat a number of infections, including sinus infections. Commonly found in tincture form, take 15 drops at a time up to three times per day.

Garlic - Garlic has properties that help fight bacteria. Overcooking deactivates the ingredient that fights bacteria, so it is best used raw. Garlic capsules are widely available.

Smoking

Smoking is an addiction, which is difficult to stop once started. Many people want to quit smoking but have a hard time. People who quit smoking suffer through many withdrawal symptoms including nervousness, irritability and insomnia. Some herbal cures are available to help make quitting easier.

Mullein - This herb helps soothe irritated lungs and mucous membranes in the respiratory tract. Take 2 to 3 cups of tea per day or ½ to 1 teaspoon of tincture three times per day.

Coltsfoot - This herb helps soothe inflamed lung tissue and also helps to loosen secretions, making it easier to cough up. Taken as a tea; drink up to 3 cups per day. Take coltsfoot for no more than four weeks per year.

Lobelia - This herb helps ease coughs and relaxes bronchial muscles. It also may help reduce nicotine cravings. Take as a mild tea, up to 3 cups daily. Lobelia has been known to cause nausea in some people so discontinue use if this happens.

Sore Throat

Many things can cause a sore throat, from postnasal drip, dry air, breathing through your mouth to a cold or virus. Antibiotics cannot treat viral infections, and left to run its course will last several days. Some herbs can soothe the symptoms of a sore throat and make it feel better.

Echinacea - Echinacea helps boost the immune system and makes it function better, and has been known to kill some viruses of the respiratory system. It can be taken along with antibiotics to treat strep throat, as it will help speed recovery. Take in capsule form. Increase the dosage at the onset of illness and decrease after several days. Do not take if you have an allergy to ragweed.

Licorice - The root of this herb helps reduce inflammation and stimulates the immune system, helping to fight infections. There are two types of licorice products. Be sure to find the licorice capsules that are for boosting the immune system and not the type used in treating ulcers.

Eucalyptus - This is a fragrant herb that soothes a sore throat. It also has antiseptic properties and can help shrink swollen tissues. It is found readily available in throat lozenges, which are a convenient way to take it. You can also drink eucalyptus tea.

Lemon Balm - Lemon balm is helpful in fighting off viruses and bacteria. Use as a tea - steep the dried leaves for 10 minutes in hot water. Strain and drink the tea warm. The tea can also be helpful when used as a gargle.

Sprains and Strained Muscles

Sprained or strained muscles may occur from overuse or exercise. Often, dehydration contributes to the sprain. Sometimes a long soak in a tub of hot water will do wonders to help replenish overused muscles. For regular sprains, apply cold packs for the first twenty-four hours after the injury. Also, keeping the injury elevated helps improve circulation and lessen the swelling. Some herbal remedies are also helpful for minor sprains and strains.

Turmeric - Turmeric has been found to have strong anti-inflammatory properties and is helpful in treating many sports injuries, including sprains. It can be used topically but is most often taken internally. Take up to 1800 milligrams per day. Do not take more, because in larger quantities it can hurt the stomach.

Kava-Kava - This herb is used to help relieve pain and as a muscle relaxant. Taken internally, you can take up to eight 500-milligram capsules per day. Do not combine kava-kava with alcohol or sedatives.

Peppermint - The cooling sensation of the peppermint helps take away from the sensation of pain, helping to feel better. Use topically for a sprain. It is available as an ingredient in many commercial creams found at the health food store. You can also use peppermint oil added to massage oil to massage into the skin.

Comfrey - Comfrey helps relieve pain, reduce swelling and inflammation. It is found in many over the counter salves and creams. It is effective without the side effects of many prescription medications. Apply as directed on the label.

Stress

Stress is unavoidable in our busy world. You can limit the amount of everyday stress you have by developing calming methods and through exercise. Some stress is dealt with through prescription medication. Herbal treatments can be very beneficial, but consult with your physician first if you are already taking medication.

Siberian Ginseng – This herb helps boost the health of the adrenal glands, helping the body resist stress-related illnesses. It can also improve mental alertness. It is safe to be used as part of a daily regime. Take in capsule form following the directions.

Panax Ginseng - This type of ginseng improves the body's ability to cope with stress. Used as a tonic, it is thought of as a fortification tonic. It is most often taken in capsule form. Herbal practitioners recommend using for two weeks at a time followed by a one-week rest before starting again. Do not take if you have high blood pressure, and do not combine with caffeine.

Schisandra - Commonly used in traditional Chinese medicine, these berries can be used as a general tonic that helps counter stress and fatigue. It also helps increase mental function. Take up to six 580-milligram capsules per day.

Kava-Kava - The root of this herb helps calm nerves without side effects associated with prescription medication. It is typically used in capsule form. Do not take with prescription drugs or alcohol, and do not drive while taking this herb as it acts like a sedative.

St.-John's-Wort - A common treatment for anxiety and depression, it is also useful in treating the symptoms of stress. Studies have shown that it is as effective as Prozac and other anti-depressants. It is commonly taken as a tea and is also available in capsule form. Do not take with prescription anti-depressants unless instructed to do so by a doctor.

Sunburn and Minor Burns

Sunburn and minor burns respond well to topical herbal treatments with salves, creams and ointments. If the burn is severe or covers a large part of the body you should seek medical treatment.

Aloe - Aloe is the best topical herbal treatment for minor burns, including sunburn. It has properties that not only cool the skin but promote fast healing. It can be readily found in any drug store. Look for aloe gel that contains close to 100% aloe.

Tea - Green and black teas act as topical cooling agents for sunburn. It has been used as a home remedy for years. Wet the tea bag with cool water and apply to the affected areas. For larger areas you can steep a kettle of tea, cool and pour over the skin as a rinse.

Calendula - Calendula is known for its anti-inflammatory and antiseptic properties. It helps cool and calm the skin, and you can use it as a tea-rinse for the skin. It is also found as a major ingredient in many herbal sunburn or skin creams found at the health food store.

Witch Hazel - Witch hazel is an astringent and acts to decrease swelling, and it also soothes the skin. Simply apply to the affected skin with a clean cloth or cotton ball.

Toothaches

A toothache can bring sever pain. It signals a problem with a tooth or gum and needs to be looked at by a dentist. If you can't get to a dentist immediately, however, you can help ease the pain with an herbal remedy.

Clove - Clove essential oil is a strong natural pain reliever. Used topically, buy clove essential oil at the health food store. Apply with a clean cloth or hold on the effected tooth with a cotton swab. Hold on for a few minutes, and it will gently numb the area.

Turmeric - This spice is known as an anti-inflammatory and antibacterial, and it helps fight infection. You can mix the spice with water to form a paste and dab onto the tooth.

Chamomile - Chamomile will help soothe the aching tooth and calm your nerves as well. It is known to fight infection and promotes healing. It is very safe to use. Drink as a tea or use the tea as a mouth rinse.

Ulcers

Ulcers are sores in the stomach or gastrointestinal tract, and they can be extremely painful. Get medical attention to determine the exact cause of the pain. Herbal treatments are useful for ulcers that are not severe.

Licorice - Herbalists say that licorice works as well on ulcers as prescription medication, but without any side effects. It helps rid the body of harmful bacteria and induces healing. Look for the form of licorice called DGL, which is the best type to use on ulcers. It needs saliva to activate the helpful ingredients, so this herb is best taken as a tea or tincture. Your use should be limited to 6 weeks at a time unless instructed otherwise by a doctor.

Chamomile - The calming properties of chamomile help heal the stomach and digestive tract. It decreases inflammation, and can also help calm nerves that perpetuate ulcers. Take as a tea or tincture up to 4 times per day.

Calendula - Calendula helps promote healing and has astringent properties that can help stop bleeding. Take as a tea or tincture up to 4 times per day.

Meadowsweet - This herb soothes the stomach and digestive tract. It reduces excess acid by soothing the stomach lining. It is available as a tea, and you should not use if you have an allergy to aspirin.

Warts

Warts are caused by a virus called the human papillomavirus, which has many strains. Common on the hands, they can pop up anywhere, especially on the face, feet and neck. You may want to try an herbal remedy to help remove warts. Remember that it can takes weeks to see any results from herbal use.

Celandine - The sap from this member of the poppy family can help reduce or eliminate warts, and helps with other skin problems as well. If you have the plant, take some of the sap and dab it onto the wart daily. If not, you can brew some strong tea with the dried root and dab the mixture onto the wart daily.

Black Birch Bark - The bark from the black birch contains antiviral compounds and salicylic acid, the same ingredients found in many over the counter wart removal salves. You can purchase the powder from a natural health store and make a paste by mixing some with water. Apply daily to the wart.

Bloodroot - This herb is known to help heal warts and has been used for centuries. Get the powder form from a natural health food store, and mix with water to form a paste and apply to the wart daily.

Dandelion - Some people claim the milk from a dandelion can remove warts. To try, simply pick the dandelion at the bottom and squeeze some of the milky inner substance onto the wart. Repeat daily.

CHAPTER 4- HERBAL RECIPES

Do not take more than the recommended dosage of an herbal product, even if it does not seem to work

It's fun and easy to make your own herbal mixtures. Many of the ingredients can be found in the kitchen, and essential oils are often found at your local natural food or supply store. If you can't find the ingredients locally there are numerous Internet stores that supply herbal oils and loose herbs.

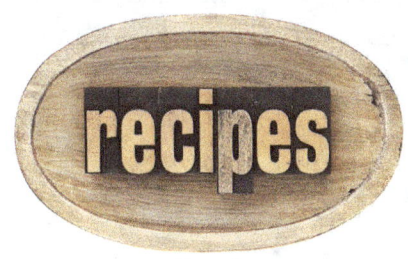

How to Make Tea

Using loose herbs to make tea is easier than it sounds. You usually use about 1 to 2 teaspoons of herbs per cup of water. Take the loose herbs and add them to a cup of hot water. Let steep for 10 minutes, and then remove the herbs. There are also special tea balls that can be used. Just put the herbs into the tea ball and immerse in hot water.

Skin Toner

Ingredients include:

Grapefruit seed extract
Witch Hazel, and
Apple cider vinegar

A wonderful skin toner can be made from Grapefruit seed extract. Mix 5 drops of grapefruit seed extract with ¼ Cup witch hazel and ½ cup apple cider vinegar together in a container. Use as a toner; after you wash your face. The toner helps keep your skin tight and helps close the pores after washing.

Canker Sore Swab

Ingredients:

2 teaspoons of Echinacea tincture
2 teaspoons of goldenseal tincture
1 teaspoon of calendula tincture
1 teaspoon of grapefruit seed extract, and
1 Tablespoon of aloe vera gel

Mix all ingredients together in a small jar, and seal tightly with a lid. To use, place a small amount on the end of a cotton swab and hold in the mouth against the sore. Hold for 5 minutes, and repeat as needed.

Cold and Flu Tea

Ingredients:

¼ Cup each dried lemon balm leaves, dried peppermint leaves, dried yarrow leaves and dried elder flowers.

Mix the dry ingredients and store in an airtight container. To mix a cup of tea, use two teaspoons of the dried herb mixture. Steep in one cup of hot water for 10 minutes, and remove the herbs. Add lemon and honey to add flavor.

Clean Scalp Hair Rinse

Ingredients:

2 Cups of apple cider vinegar, and
¼ Cup dried sage, rosemary or thyme leaves (alone or in any combination)

Heat the apple cider vinegar to boiling and remove from heat. Add the herbs and cover for 10 minutes. Strain the mixture, leaving only the liquid. Put the mixture into a container (an old shampoo bottle will work great) and use each time you wash your hair. To use, mix with water as you rinse your hair with it. This helps control dandruff.

Swimmer's Drops

Ingredients:

¼ Cup Vinegar
¼ Cup rubbing alcohol, and
2 –3 drops of grapefruit extract, garlic tincture or Echinacea tincture

Sterilize a small glass bottle. Mix the ingredients in the bottle and cap tightly. To use, put 1–3 drops into the ear with an eyedropper, and allow to run out.

Eyestrain Teabags

Use these teabags to help soothe tired eyes, as well as to help you relax.

Make a strong herbal tea infusion using your choice of herbs. Steep the herbs in hot water for 10 minutes, and strain the liquid. Soak a clean cotton cloth in the liquid and squeeze the excess out. Close your eyes and place the cloth on your closed eyelids for 10 minutes. This feels best when still warm.

Homemade Cough Syrup

This can be used to treat mild coughs due to colds. Take ½ teaspoon every two to three hours.

Ingredients:

½ Cup Water
½ Cup Honey, and
5 teaspoons of dried herbs – any combination of the following herbs: Mullein leaves, horehound, rosemary leaves, cinnamon bark, ginger, cayenne.

Combine the ingredients in a pot on the stove and bring to a boil. Simmer until the mixture reduces to about half. Then, remove and strain the herbs, leaving only the liquid. Cool and pour into a small glass container, and store in the refrigerator.

Toothache Compound

If you can't get to the dentist right away, try this homemade toothache remedy. It will help keep the tooth from becoming infected as well as keep the pain down.

Ingredients:

1 drop clove bud essential oil

2 drops German chamomile essential oil, and

½ teaspoon goldenseal powder

Mix all ingredients together to form a paste, and apply to the effected tooth with a cotton swab. Use up to 4 times per day.

CONCLUSION

Most herbal remedies are safe; in fact, in most cases they have few or no side effects. They are a natural alternative to treating conditions. While many herbal remedies are safe, it is important to understand that there are some risks involved in using them. In order to be safe, follow these guidelines when using herbal remedies.

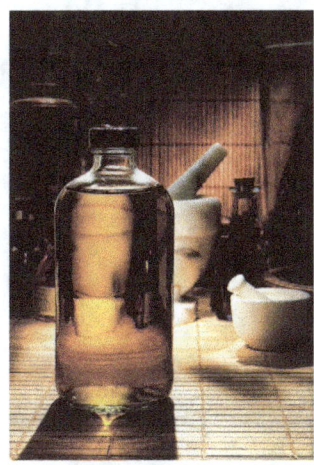

Interactions between herbal remedies and prescription drugs can occur. Read the directions that come with any pre-made herbal remedies that you buy.

Do not stop taking prescription drugs unless you first check with your doctor. Some prescriptions are necessary in keeping certain problems under control, such as heart disease and high blood pressure.

If you are under a doctor's care, meet with him to tell him you want to start taking herbal remedies. Together you can come up with a plan that will work for your specific circumstance.

If you are pregnant, do not take any herbal remedies without first consulting with your doctor.

Do not take more than the recommended dosage of an herbal product, even if it does not seem to work. Not all herbal remedies work the same on all people. Also, some herbal remedies need to build up in the system over days or weeks before they become effective.

Do not use herbal remedies on children under 3 without the approval of their doctor.

When giving herbal remedies to children, remember to give the correct dosage for their weight. Do not give too much to a child.

Start with the lowest recommended dosage for your condition. If needed, you can increase the dose later on. When using skin creams you should test them on a small patch of unaffected skin first, to make sure you are not allergic to anything in them.

ABOUT THE AUTHOR

It's amazing how much we can do in natural ways to make our bodies feel better. I didn't get into or consider body detoxification or herbal remedies until I got sick and just got tired of taking pills. I wanted an alternative to make me feel better if I came down with something. Or even if I didn't come down with something, I wanted to keep my body healthy all the time, if possible.

A friend of mine turned me on to taking care of my body without prescriptions the way that she does and I totally got hooked on taking an interest in anything natural. This eventually led up to me wanting to share the things I knew with others by writing about it so that they too can feel better not only physically, but mentally as well because our mind and body goes hand in hand.

After you take in the information and put it into practice, you'll see just how great for your health taking a natural path really is.

www.ingramcontent.com/pod-product-compliance
Lightning Source LLC
Chambersburg PA
CBHW081244280526
45787CB00006B/2789